BREAK THROUGH
WEIGHT LOSS
5 Proven Ways to Get and Stay Healthy,

Today!

By
Todd Stocker

Published by

Cannon River Press

IMPORTANT: Before you dive into any change in your diet or exercise routine, consult your health advisor or physician! In fact, bring this book with you to let them know how you are going to be able to change your life! Results vary per person.

TABLE OF CONTENTS

Begin Today!

Most weight loss books and programs are all the same. In fact, you could probably state the two things that everyone says are the keys to losing weight and getting healthy. Say them with me, "Eat right" and "exercise." The problem is that you've been there and done that. You've tried all the advice. You've counted the points and the calories. You've bought the food scales and the portion bowls and yet, you find yourself mildly to severely overweight.

My message to you is:

THERE IS HOPE!

My Story

I am not a licensed trainer or nutritionalist. I don't hold degrees in physical fitness or health therapy. I am simply an everyday person, like you, who has always struggled with being overweight but has learned some Break Through techniques that have helped me lose 40 pounds in 3 months!

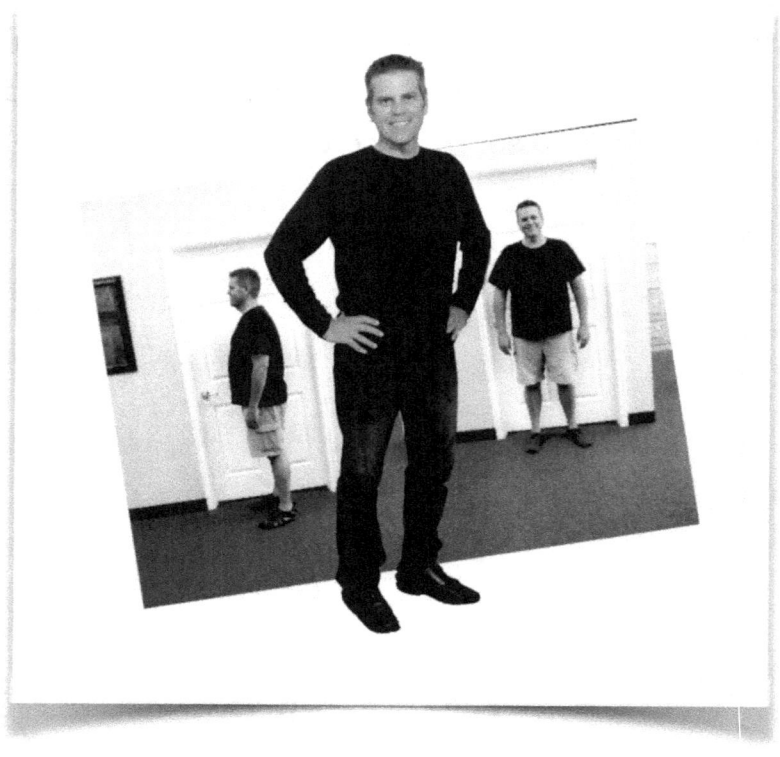

My mom always told me that our family is "big-boned" which I never understood (although there is some truth to what she was saying). I was called the chubby kid in school which meant that I was relegated to always being last when the kids picked out their teams. In fact, my nickname all through grade school was "Taco" because, as they said, I had all the fillings. I know. Kids can be mean.

Fast forward to high school and into college where my natural growth curve slimmed me out a bit with also slimmed away my low self-esteem. This resulted in a sense of confidence and joy which helped me find a girlfriend and eventually a wife. Soon after the honeymoon, however, the pounds started piling up again. Then, some in my heavyset family had the dreaded bariatric surgery and I watched them physically be forced to only eat tablespoons of food at a time. YUCK! At about that time, I went into my doctor for an annual check up and he told me that I was "obese."

I don't know if you've ever been labeled that before but for me, it hurt, even more than the name calling in grade school. So my wife and I decided to get healthy. We tried Atkins. We tried counting calories. We tried skipping meals, juicing, vegetable diets, soup diets and even switching dinner for breakfast (which I loved doing, by the way).

We lost a few pounds here and there but nothing significant and we always felt like we were depriving ourselves of the food and drink that we've come to enjoy.

Then a few months ago, I interview Lisa Rambo. She was a contestant on the TV show "The Biggest Loser" — season 14. She is an amazing woman who lost 108 pounds and has kept it off! (You can see her journey by going to her Facebook page — http://on.fb.me/15SOMnr.) She inspired me to at least begin thinking about getting healthy again.

Finally, on July 1st, my wife and I had a "Popeye" moment. We looked at ourselves in the mirror and said together, "That's all I can stands, I can't stands no more!" With that, we made a conscious decision to get healthy.

Since that time, we've both lost a 5 year old (in terms of weight), are biking 20 miles without breaking a sweat and recently completed our first Triathlon! That was when I was only half way through of my weight loss journey! Never saw that coming!

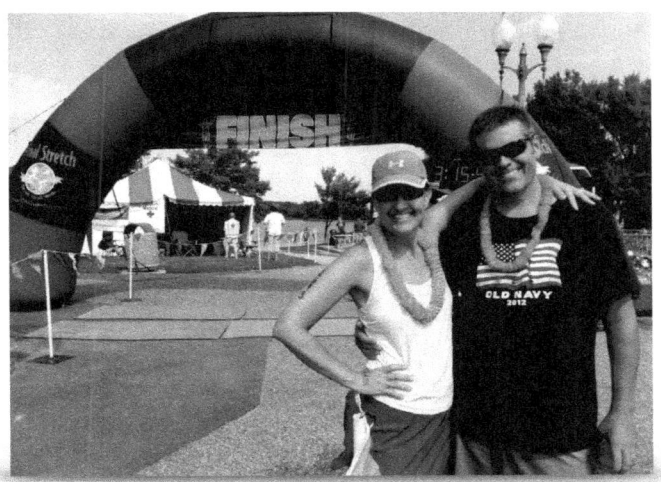

I have more energy, more focus and can bounce back quicker than before from those times when negative feelings seem to pound against emotional castle.

Here are my stats so far. I started my journey at 231 pounds. Today I'm at 191. My goal is 185 which gives me a 5 pound "bumper zone" based on my height and age. I've gone from a 40 inch waist to 34 inch and I'm feeling great! In fact, here is a chart how my weight loss has gone, week by week.

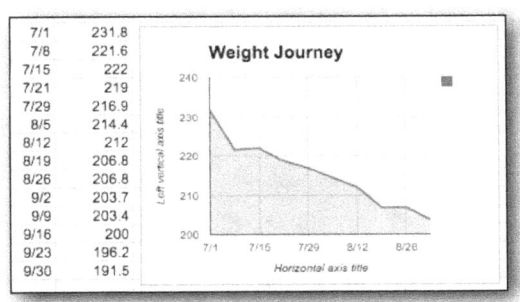

Notice that at the beginning, I lost more pounds faster and slower as I'm leveling out into my goal weight. This is normal and it will be for you.

Now I know that these numbers aren't incredible. In fact you can see some plateaus and weight gains along the way. So while it's not spectacular, it doesn't take spectacular changes to make your life better!

As I write this book, I want you to know that I've been where you are right now and it wasn't that long ago. I am not that different from you. I will gain some of my weight back and will bounce around based on my emotions and events. But this book is not about becoming the next Albert Schweitzer, Jack Lalanne, Tony Horton or The Rock. It is about you and me — everyday people who want to get and be healthy, long term.

What you're going to absorb in the next "pages" are some of my learnings as I've struggled with my weight and how I finally have broken through to lifelong health. **Whether you want to lose 10 pounds or 50, this book can help you get there!**

Again …

YOU CAN DO IT!
YOU CAN BREAK THROUGH!

Summary

In this chapter, I told my story of Break Through and how you can do it as well. In fact, this book will give you the same principles and Break Throughs that I used to lose weight and get healthy.

On another note, on average, women can lose 3-5 pounds per week while men can lose 5-7 pounds a week.

Get Your Head On Straight

Most of us become unhealthy because of feelings. While some of us do have medical conditions, a great majority of us are driven to "feel better" about ourselves or our circumstances and so we turn to immediate gratification to ease the pain. I was one. I ate to feel better. I mean, who could deny that a pepperoni and mushroom pizza at midnight would quell the pain of any romantic breakup! I know, right!

Before you begin any journey, it is important to get your head in the right place. Visualize the journey on which your are going to embark. If you are a spiritual person, this is when you spend an extended time alone in prayer, asking God for strength. Make sure that you set yourself up for success by mentally making the choice to do this. But you can't do it alone.

Hiking Partners

If you think you can do this without the help of others YOU WILL FAIL. Sorry, but it's true. There is no way that I am strong enough to slowly change an eating pattern that has developed over decades without my wife's help.

This is when you find one to three people — no more — to be your "hiking partners" to help encourage you in the journey. Be open with them. For me, it was my wife, a few friends and family and some professional partners (see the end of the book). We are doing the journey together. They are my encouragers and my teachers. If you don't have a significant other, ask a friend or co-worker. There are three criteria to find these other people:

1) They have to be trusted.

You have to know that what you share with them isn't going to be posted on FaceBook or blabbed in casual conversation. This is why healthcare professionals are important on your list of hiking partners.

2) They must to have a balance of concern. for you.

There are some people you know who would be calling you at midnight wondering if you're eating the late-night ice cream. They are the crazies. On the other extreme are people who never ask you the hard questions. You need people who can balance both. It may even be your Pastor or spiritual leader.

3) They need to have a positive attitude.

The demons in your psyche are going to have a field day when you embark on this adventure. They will point their finger at you when the scale goes up instead of down. They will tell you that you can't do it and that you are weak so you need people around you who can give real perspective that leans in a positive direction.

Right now, think of one person who would match a few of the above characteristics. Write that person's name down. Now the hard part: Call them and invite them to help you. You can do it. I'd also like to be one of your hiking partners. Just connect with me at www.TheLifeShoppe.com and let me know about your journey. Confidentially, I'll send you encouragements along the way.

What do you want to gain?

One of my "hiking partners" asked me a fantastic question before I began my weight loss adventure. He asked, "At the end of this journey, what is it that you want to *gain*?" That question forced me to look at the positive side of something I've battled my whole life. That question repositions weight loss as a means to an end. You don't lose weight just to lose weight or avoid heart attacks. You lose weight for the benefits that you gain!

For me, I wanted to gain comfort. I am a public speaker and so I stand in front of many people at a time. I wanted to feel comfortable in the clothes I was wearing and comfortable knowing that I looked and felt good.

As you begin, write down what it is you want to gain rather than lose. Some people write down "confidence," others put down "energy" and still others have written "time." Many people have written down "a spouse."

Be honest with yourself. Visualize yourself 10, 30, or 50 pounds lighter. What would that look like *internally* not just *externally*?

Now, it is okay to occasionally think about what you're going to lose as well. Some of those loses are weight, shame, guilt, depression and so on. For me, I jokingly said that I want to lose the 'X' in my 'XL'. I've done that and more!

One last tip on the mental part of your upcoming Break Through. If you don't do something now, what will your life look like in 6 months? Marcus Buckingham (http://amzn.to/18SDTOE) wrote a thought in one of his books that said, "Play out your life like a movie." The idea being that if nothing changes, how will the movie of your life end? That scared me because, as I mentioned before, several in my family struggle with health and I could see myself ending the same way.

Above all, remember that you were created as a masterpiece. For you, there is some discovering that needs to happen but the masterpiece is in you. Don't get down on yourself. You are valuable and have high worth in your Creators heart. Remember ...

YOU CAN DO IT!

YOU CAN BREAK THROUGH!

Summary

In this chapter, I discussed the important first step of mentally choosing to get healthy. I also said that having a small group of "hiking partners" is key to your success as well.

1)   Find people who will share this journey with you.

2)   Focus on what you want to gain, not what you will lose.

3) Play out in your mind what life could look like 3 months from now if you succeed.

The Role of Movement

I not a fan of the word *exercise*. Growing up, that word reminded me of hard workouts when I played sports which resulted in my sore knees and tentative ankles.

However, getting moving is something your body needs. So call it exercise, call it movement, they key is to take small steps toward getting your body out of a sedentary lifestyle. No matter at what level you are active, the next sections are critical to understanding your Break Through weight loss!

Flip your 80-20 thinking

I used to think that 80% of weight loss was exercise and 20% was what I ate. That is what I had experienced when I was in high school and college. But again, I was involved in high intensity sports so of course, I experienced leanness through exercise.

If you're reading this book, I'll bet that you are not as active as you once were. I'll take a second bet that you are rather sedentary for most of your day. That is how life is for most Americans anyway.

But before we address your activity you need to flip your thinking! More and more studies are proving that weight loss — long term, healthy weight loss — is 80% nutrition and 20% exercise! I use to run miles and miles and only lose a few pounds here and there. But since learning and applying the 80-20 flip rule, I have seen incredible results!

We'll talk about food and drink intake in the next Break Through chapters but I want to make sure you are hearing me correctly.

I am NOT saying that you should stop moving.

You need to be moving/exercising consistently! You need to be part of a workout facility that has your health as its top priority! Movement is still a key part of getting healthy. Movement is what makes you strong. Combined with correct eating and drinking, it gives you more energy. Movement also enhances chemicals that make you feel happy which is key to making these Break Through's work for you.

Here is what I mean by movement. Movement is intentional action that results in an elevated heart rate. Here is what my wife and I have been doing:

Walking: We have a small park and lake by our home. So, a few times a week in the evening, we stroll and talk and before long, we've walked the 2 miles and have reconnected as a couple. We don't schedule these. It's just a natural part of what we do. You don't need to have anyone go with you. Just substitute 20 minutes of watching TV after dinner with a walk while listening to music or a podcast.

Biking: This is the activity that I love the most. Four to five times a month, I take my bike on some paths in my area and enjoy the outdoors. I bike an average of 40 minutes which isn't that difficult to do. You can have a stationary bike or go to a gym for this as well. I just love the beauty of creation and find myself getting lost in it. Once a month, I try to do a 30-40 mile ride. That's more intense so again, check with your doctor if you decide to be Lance Armstrong!

Jogging: I don't suggest this if you're severely overweight or have other medical conditions that would irritate such conditions. But for me, I have been able to jog again as my weight has dropped to a healthy level. I jog maybe once or twice a week but no more.

What activities could you be doing starting today? Take small steps in this. Maybe it's taking the stairs instead of the escalator. Maybe it's making a few trips back and forth to your car as you unload the groceries.

Notice that I'm not encouraging huge steps. Baby steps help you grow. Below are a "Baby Steps" tool that will help you identify simply ways to get moving:

1. On a piece of paper, make a list of all the things you do that would classify as "movement." (walking to and from the parking lot at work, jogging, etc.)

2. Put a star by the ones that cause you to break a sweat — even a little bit. Keep doing those!

3. Draw an up arrow by the ones that you may be able to increase in frequency or intensity. Then increase them, incrementally!

Again, this is a guide for everyday people like you and me. Athletic trainers or those training for some high intense activity will have different lists than you and me. But just this simple tool can help you get to the 20% that your body needs to be healthy.

Remember that even if you're active now, there are times in your life when you become sedentary.

Don't get down on yourself.   Don't seek to look like someone else.   The goal here is health not comparison.

In the next sections, we will dive into the 5 Break Through's that have changed my life. They are:

Just Add Water
Front Load Your Day
Eat A Lot
Weigh Everyday
Celebrate Good Times

Remind yourself that this is a journey. Some days, you'll suck at this.   Other days, you're going to feel great. But above all, remember that

YOU CAN DO IT! YOU CAN BREAK THROUGH!

Summary

In this chapter, we discussed the importance of doing some sort of movement and how to start to increase the amount.

1) Make sure you include movement in your daily activity.

2) Weight loss is 80% intake and 20% movement.

3)   Use the "Baby Steps" tool to help identify opportunities to increase your movement during your day.

Break Through 1: Just Add Water

The system through which your body expels waste, toxins and the fat that you'll be using is lubricated by water — more generally — liquids. Picture a dirty bowl. Let's say you pour a little water into it. What happens? The dirt is pulled from the side of the bowl and mixed in with the water. But if you leave the water there and it evaporates, what happens to the dirt? It ends up clinging right back to the bowl. But if, when the dirt is in the water and you pour the water out, then the dirt is gone from the bowl.

In your Break Through weight loss, the principle is the same. As your body begins to shed the unwanted fat, liquids are the vehicle into which they are transported out of your body. Pretty slick, right!

For me, I hate the taste of water. I know, water doesn't have a taste, but to my tongue, it does. So when I'm drinking water, I add a hint of lemon or lime juice to it. You can also use sugar-free additions to water to make it more palatable but try to keep as close to the original water as possible.

There are also vitamin waters on the market as well. You can drink the zero calorie ones but don't make them your main liquid intake. Simple water is the best.

Getting Specific

All researchers and nutritionists agree that water is important to any diet. In my study, I've found that they are all over the place when it comes to amounts. Here's what I've done to lose my 40 pounds (so far).

I shoot for 10 drinks a day (or 80 oz for those of you who are anal about measuring things). At the beginning, this was TORTURE! As I said before, I've never liked the taste of water so it took me a few weeks to get use to this routine. You notice that I didn't say *ounces* or anything like that. Again, if you have to take time to measure something, you'll never stick with it. So here's what I do now — my typical day. Remember that this works for me. It might not work for you.

My Daily Water In-Take

1) When I wake up, I turn on my coffee maker (yes, you can drink coffee with skim milk and a small amount of sugar-free sweetener. See Break Through #3 for suggested sweeteners). I have my first glass of water while my coffee is warming up.

2) After my cup of coffee, I full up my daily water bottle and begin sucking on that. I purchased a 24 oz water bottle - 3 drinks — from Walmart for 10 bucks and I carry it everywhere. The great thing about the recent health craze is that most of these bottles already have 8oz 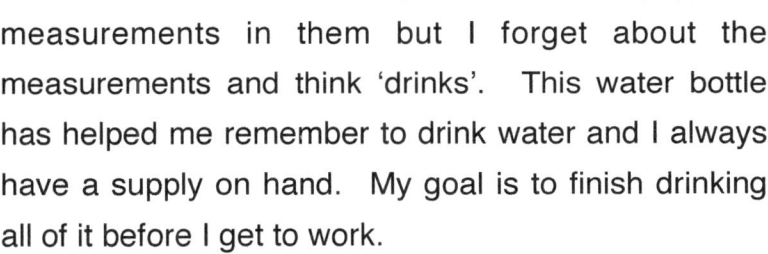 measurements in them but I forget about the measurements and think 'drinks'. This water bottle has helped me remember to drink water and I always have a supply on hand. My goal is to finish drinking all of it before I get to work.

3) When I get to work, I refill it right away along with another cup of coffee (skim milk and sugar-free sweetener as before).

4) By 10 am, I've finished my second filled water bottle. At this point, let's do a count.

Time	Drinks
6:00 am	1
8:00 am	3
10:00 am	5
Total:	7

As you can see that by 10 am, I'm more than half way to my 10 drink daily goal at 7 cups of water. Just think of all the "dirt" that is being washed from your "bowl!" Let's continue.

5) Again, I refill my bottle. It's about 10 or 11 in the morning. This time, I don't feel like I need to slam it all down. In fact, my body automatically tells me to slow down with the water in-take. From 10 am till lunch time, I sip the water as I need it or as I remind myself to.

6) By lunch or a little into the afternoon, I've finished or have come close to finishing my third bottle. The count is 9 - 10 drinks and I still have the rest of the day to go!

7) Now, I'm hitting the restroom pretty consistently which is the way it should be. (Again, think 'dirt' and 'bowl').

At this point, the rest of the day is gravy! By 3 or 4 in the afternoon, you should already be at your 10 drinks. If you are involved in heavy physical activity, make sure you keep well hydrated. 10 drinks a day may not be enough if you are involved in heavy athletics or have a job that requires you to exert energy. Consult your doctor on that.

Other Water Tips

Feeling hungry? Drink water first. Did you know that sometimes when you think you're hungry, your body may actually just be thirsty? To test it out, when you have that physical grumbling or mental craving, first drink a glass of water (flavored or straight). Wait three minutes and think about your stomach again. Your body will let you know if you need to eat something as well.

Don't go crazy on measuring! Remember, even just saying, "a glass of water" is mentally more effective than measuring exactly 8 oz. You're not drinking enough now, right? So don't worry about exact amounts. Mentally this will destroy you.

Avoid "dirty water"

Many people have asked me, "Does it need to be pure water?" "What about Diet Soda's or juices?" My typical response is, "Avoid dirty water." Dirty water is a liquid that comes in the form of something other than water. Yes, I still have a light beer, wine and scotch occasionally. Yes, I drink diet 7UP and diet Ginger-ale. But as you'll find, these simply slow-down your weight loss.

For me, I generally don't like the taste of plain water so I'll add lemon juice to it which no only helps the taste, but also increases the alkalinity. Without getting too technical, an increased alkalinity helps with digestion and weight loss. So you have to ask yourself, "How fast to I want to Break Through to my weight loss goal?"

What About Alcohol?

I saved this one for a special category because I enjoy beer, wine and scotch and I still drink them on my Break Through. Below are the primary questions I get regarding alcohol:

1) Can I drink alcohol?

Yes, just remember that it's dirty water and will slow down your weight loss. If you have alcohol daily, forget about weight loss. You plateau and begin gaining again.

2) How much can I drink?

My rule of thumb has been, *"One is fun; Two and I'm done."* This is a great place for your hiking partners to come in. They can help you keep accountable on this.

3) Specifically, what adult beverage can I drink?

Beer: I'm a hoppy-beer guy, but they have a lot of calories. During your Break Through weight loss phase, limit yourself to a light beer. I know, the taste may suck. Try added a dash of salt into the beer. It spruces up the flavor and brings out some of the taste. During my phase, I drank Lite Beer from Miller, Amstel Light, Miller 64, and Mic Ultra Amber.

Wine: There is a line of low-calorie wine called 'Skinny Girl'. It's not bad and satisfies your taste. After about week three, your metabolism can handle a normal two-glass wine event without a hiccup. But remember the phrase, *"One is fun; Two and I'm done."*

Spirits: As mentioned before, I'm a scotch drinker. Just remember that scotch and other spirits have consolidated calories, meaning that the servings are typically smaller but still have as much if not more that a typical beer or wine.

Here is a calorie comparison website that's pretty interesting but ignore the title. I do not and will never advocate for anyone to get drunk: http://getdrunknotfat.com.

First Step

Don't feel overwhelmed. Don't adjust anything else in your diet yet. Simply try this for 3 or 4 days and see what happens. I'll bet you dollars to donuts that you begin losing weight and you'll begin feeling better physically and emotionally. It will take a while to get use to but remember that ...

YOU CAN DO IT!

YOU CAN BREAK THROUGH!

Summary

In this chapter, we discussed the importance of adding water to your diet.

1. Buy a water bottle from Walmart and keep it filled all day long.

2. Think 'drinks' rather than ounces or even cups.

3. Try to drink as close to original water as possible, adding lemon or sugar-free dink mixes if needed.

4. When you feel hungry, drink a glass of water first. Your body might be thirsty rather than hungry.

5. Certain alcohol is permitted but in moderation. Remember the phrase "One is fun; Two and I'm done."

Break Through 2: Front Load Your Day

Go back to Break Through 1 and notice that most of my water intake happened before 3 pm. That's what it means to front load. Simply put, the amount you eat and drink during the day should be weighted more heavily in the morning and early afternoon than later or into the evening.

Let me explain your body. The first meal of the day, in most cultures, is called "breakfast." The reason is that it *breaks the fast* that your body has been in for the last 6-8 hours. When your mind wakes up, it signals your body to wake up as well and begin moving. In order for it to do that, your body looks for nourishment to being fueling itself to accomplish daily living — whatever that looks like in its context. In other words, your brain needs to feed the machine called your body. If your body isn't given its fuel at the beginning and middle of the day, it thinks that you are in the Sahara Dessert and will begin preparing for a long journey of "non-fuel." This is simply a survival technique that our Creator designed in us.

When your body goes into this kind of starvation-mode, as nutritionists call it, it begins to store fat for the long Sahara-Dessert trip. That's why not eating does not help you lose fat. I'll talk about that more in Break Through #3.

So when you try to eat and drink your daily goals up front (front loading), your body kicks into gear and begins burning the extra fat because it knows that the fuel to do so is being supplied.

By 3 or 4 in the afternoon, you should have taken in most of your daily drinking and eating goals. For me, this took some adjusting because I struggle with the late afternoon munchies. Don't worry! I'll discuss that more in Break Through 3!

Here's a funny story from my childhood that relates to front loading. My mom tried it with our family. She switched the breakfast menu with the dinner menu. So when I woke up, I would smell hamburgers, pizza and spaghetti being prepared. This caused a full and happy tummy as I ventured off to school. When I came home, we'd sit down to bacon and eggs, cereal or pancakes. I loved it! However, my mom was so tired of waking up at 5 in the morning to prepare dinner, after one week she quit. Too bad. I loved the switch!

Remember that ...

YOU CAN DO IT!

YOU CAN BREAK THROUGH!

Summary

In this chapter, we discussed how your body cycles through food. It is best to eat and drink most of your daily in take by 3 or 4 in the afternoon. That gives your body plenty of calories for your daily activities and speeds up your metabolism.

Break Through 3: Eat A Lot

(This is the longest chapter in the book because there is so much to share. However, I boiled it down to very manageable information. You may want to keep this chapter handy as you begin to adjust your eating patterns).

Over the years, my weight loss and getting healthy journey has been an up and down road. I know it is for you as well or you wouldn't be reading this book. I would get on a health craze and hit all the trendy diets. You know the ones. Their titles describe parts of the country, something someone did in the Bible or they use the words, "Quick" or "Fast." From my experience, they all have ideas that are helpful but do you really learn anything? Can you maintain it after a few weeks, months or even years?

What I've been learning and doing isn't a diet. It's a way of managing 'when' and 'what' of your intake to maximize this incredible body machine in which you live. Unlike juicing or non-carb intake, I believe that these Break Throughs are not a one-time shot. For me, I'll be able to settle into a comfortable weight and live the rest of my days in a healthy state - God willing.

So here's what I've learned about eating in Break Through number three and it will help you fire up your metabolism, lose the weight and look and feel incredible. There are three "Don'ts" that I just want to get out of the way.

1) Don't skip a meal.

You read that right. Don't skip a meal. Remember the Sahara Dessert conversation in Break Through 2? If you skip a meal, your body could go into "starvation mode" and you'll actual negatively impact your health and you'll gain weight with the next meal.

I know. It doesn't make sense. I always thought that if I skip a meal I'm not taking in calories and I'll lose weight. It is true that you'll be taking in less calories, but in starvation mode, your body will hoard the next meal you eat. It will almost immediately turn it into fat, thinking that it needs to store it for the Sahara Dessert. (I really should visit that place. But I digress).

I've been eating 3 meals a day and 2-3 snacks a day. Yes! You can snack in your new Break Through lifestyle! It is a lot of food and sometimes I can't even eat all of it. But I am more satisfied now and don't have those killer cravings *as much* anymore.

2) Don't eat Fake Food.

It's not rocket science. The basic formula is:

Food - Fake Food = Break Through Weight Loss and Health

Food: Everything in your fridge, cabinets and glove compartment of your car that you eat because you're hungry, bored, stimulated, impulsive, happy or sad.   Basically, anything you put in your mouth and digest through your system.

Fake Food: Anything that is 30% or more processed. What is processed food? Any food that has been prepared mainly for ease of convenience or use.   They usually contain an overage of preservatives and sodium to make their "shelf life" last forever.

- Prepared mixes (pancake or cake mix)
- Frozen foods (vegetables, pizza)
- Processed Cheese (most store-bought cheese)
- Canned food (beans, Tuna in oil)
- Snack food (bagged chips, pretzels)
- Certain Breads (anything with white flour, usually and some whole wheat breads as well)
- Fast food (to avoid a lawsuit, I'm not going to list them but you know who they are).   There are some

healthy options at such places, however. I list some of them in a later section.

You get the idea.

But before you stop reading, you CAN have processed food. You just need to know that it slows down and can even reverse your Break Through weight loss. That is such a key understanding that I want to repeat it and highlight it …

If you eat off-plan, it simply slows down your weight loss.

This is important to know, especially when I talk about "Grace Time" in a following chapter. Anyway, I'll prove this truth. Let's go back to the chart of my weight loss.

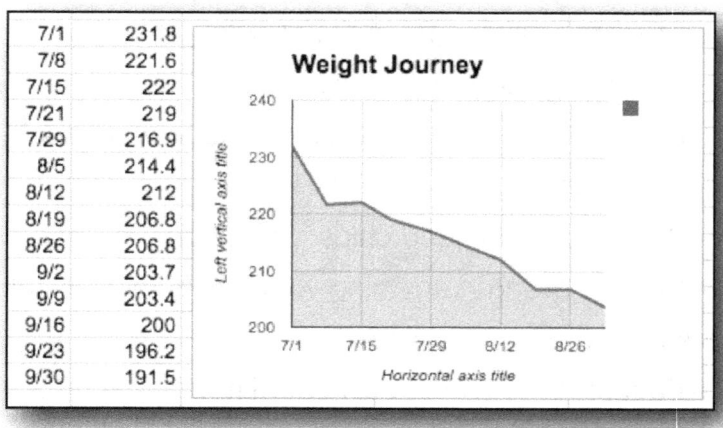

7/1	231.8
7/8	221.6
7/15	222
7/21	219
7/29	216.9
8/5	214.4
8/12	212
8/19	206.8
8/26	206.8
9/2	203.7
9/9	203.4
9/16	200
9/23	196.2
9/30	191.5

Weight Journey

On 8/25, right before the chart shows my weigh in on the 26th, I ate pizza with my kids resulting in a slow down that week — actually a stall. On 9/2, I had two hotdogs after a running event. If that's not processed, I don't know what is!

The key is to try to eat food that is closest to its original state. While I love beef jerky, real beef is better for me. Dried salmon is awesome but grilled over open flame is much better. Jack LaLanne, one of the original fitness guru's who lived to be 97 years old always said:

"If God didn't make it, I don't eat it."
Jack LaLanne

If you've made the decision to follow these Break Throughs and you have a bag of Doritos, don't quit what you've started! Just because you fall of the proverbial "wagon" doesn't mean you are left in the dust. You are not a bad person. You are not a failure! Failure is simply and event and not a label. Just be aware that it will slow down your weight loss and journey to health. Again, I talk more about this in the section called Grace Time.

3) Don't skimp on the right food.

If I had to measure everything into portions and weights, I would not be healthy today. Our lives are too busy for that. If you want to follow a program that counts points and meters, that's totally up to you. For me, I don't carry around a chart or have a calorie counter app. I'm too busy. So, for the Break Through weight loss, here's the saying:

"FIST SIZE IS THE RIGHT SIZE"

Your stomach, in it's natural state, is about fist size. Go ahead and make a fist right now. It can expand to greater sizes than that but it is roughly that size. Some diets say that you should only eat that much IN TOTAL. However, there is research that says your stomach works best when it is moderately stretched during your intact to create and excrete enzymes that facilitate digestion. Basically, use "FIST SIZE IS THE RIGHT SIZE" for the components of a Break Through meal.

There are 5 components of a Break Through Weight Loss Meal.

1) Protein.
2) Vegetable.

3) Fruit.

4) Starch.

5) Liquids.

1) **Protein**

I'm a meat guy. I love beef, chicken, seafood. So when I found that I could still eat meat and lose weight, I was pumped! There are meats to avoid during your Break Through weight loss phase. Mainly pork. Unfortunately, pork has a high fat content over and above healthier options so stay away from them.

But protein isn't just meat. Dairy products also count as protein as well as eggs and tofu.

In every meal, your protein can consist of <u>one</u> of the following:

* Eggs: Chicken eggs are the easiest. This is the one exception to the "FIST SIZE IS THE RIGHT SIZE" rule. To make a fist-sized pile of eggs is too much. Just one or two will do it.

* Cottage cheese: I enjoy this occasionally for breakfast with a dash of light salt and pepper.

* Beef: Try to stick with the leaner options. Most packaging gives a percentage of lean. Don't eat Beef everyday because it takes longer to digest. Three times per week is plenty.

* Poultry: The two I eat most are chicken and turkey. AVOID the fake-food processed stuff. (see number 2 above)

* Fish and Shellfish: Tuna in water, shrimp, tilapia are all good.

2) Vegetable

Vegetables are the one thing you can eat as much as you want, whenever you want. I call them "open-fisted" food because there really isn't a limit. Asparagus, Cauliflower, Celery, Mushrooms, Snow Peas—they all count. Basically, anything you pull out of the ground is fair game. But don't stir fry them up in butter and sauces. That's where your Break Through weight loss will slow down.

3) Fruit

Fruit helps stimulate your metabolism and provides the needed sugars for your body. According to www.energyfiend.com, one apple has the same amount of sugar as half a can of Coke. The difference is that it is a natural sugar. Contrary to a popular belief, apples do not contain caffeine but fruit, in general can give you a sugar rush because their fructose is digested quickly. Along with apples, blueberries, cherries, grapefruit, kiwi, oranges and watermelon are all on the list.   Make sure to implement the "FIST SIZE IS THE RIGHT SIZE" rule.   Too much of even natural sugar can make you feel sick.

4) Starch

This one was the most difficult for me to grasp.   To me, starch was something I wanted in my dry-cleaned shirts.   But starches are in the same family as carbohydrates or breads.   Of all the items on which your body might have trouble cutting back, it is carbs. Carbohydrates are essential to your body but the wrong carbs can slow down your Break Through weight loss.

Health expert Kyle Leon (http://on.fb.me/ 1bspC01), says that when you're younger, your body can process carbs at a faster rate than when you're older.   He suggests that starting at the age of 21, you should slowly decrease your carb intake and replace them with healthier options like starches.

Starches are a simpler form of carbs and help with the digestive process.   This portion of your meal is a bit more difficult to come by.   You may have to go to a specialty food store for some items.

Some examples of the starches that I eat are 1 slice of diet (whole grain) bread, an unsalted rice cake, half of a corn tortilla, small baked potato, or a plain gluten-free cracker. Run a Google search to get a more complete list if you'd like.

Go easy on these.

5) Liquids

Unless you have trouble swallowing food as you eat it, try to drink your liquids toward the end of your meal. Research shows that liquids can wash away the enzymes needed to breakdown food as it enters the digestive system. So holding off with allow these enzymes to do their work on your food before they're washed away.

As I mentioned in the section on drinking water, I'd stick with water during your meals. You want your body to be concentrating on process your "food" not your "drink" during that time but that's up to you. It is okay to have one cup of skim milk a day however (yes, I know. Skim milk takes a bit to get use to but if you drink it ice cold, it's not bad). For other beverages, see Break Through 1.

Here is a typical Breakfast, Lunch and Dinner for me (actually this was from today). I also had grapes before this lunch picture so they aren't in there. I added milk and a diet clear soda to show you that you can drink these as well. However, I normally just drink water

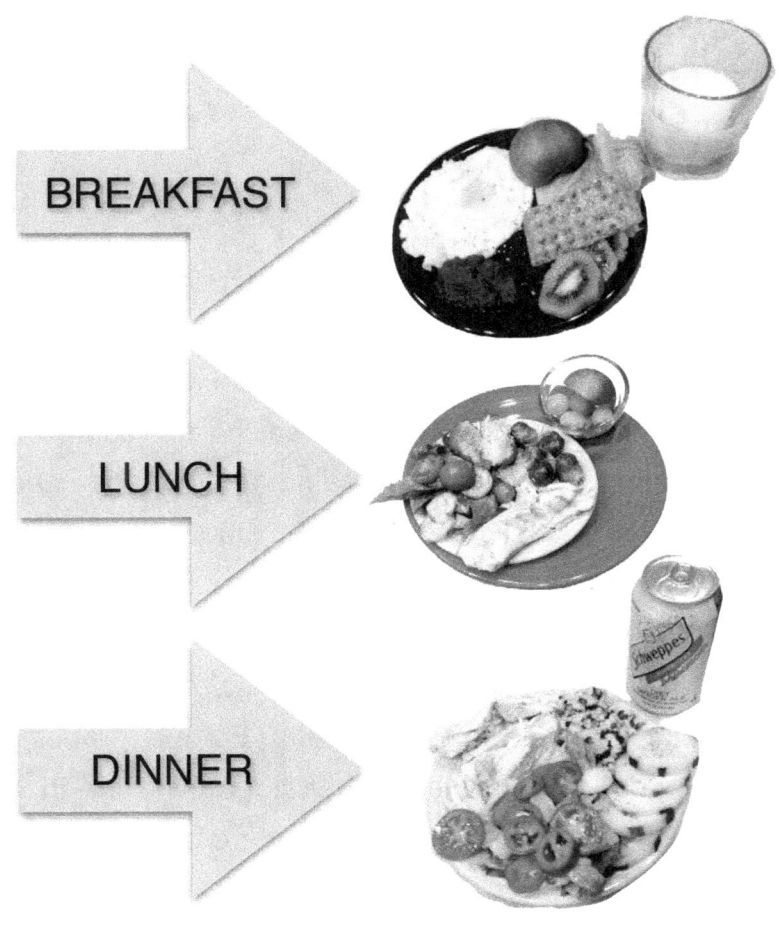

Make sure you snack!

So here's my daily schedule. I don't follow it minute by minute but I've learned that my body works best on this schedule. As you learn more about your body's health patterns, you may have to adjust it.

7am   - Breakfast

10am   - Snack

12:30pm - Lunch

3:00pm   - Snack

5 or 6pm - Dinner

8pm   - Small Snack (sometimes)

As you can see, it's not rocket science.   The healthcare industry has been saying the same thing for years. Every two to three hours, your body needs some kind of intake to keep the fires of your metabolism burning.

What kind of snack should you eat? If you've read this far, you could probably say it already.   A snack that is closest to its natural state. For me, grabbing a nectarine or a low-cal, natural protein bar in the morning is the best because they are portable. Other vegetables and fruits also are good. Just make sure your snacks are low-calorie. If I'm buying a packaged snack, I make sure they are around 100 calories or so and not FAKE-FOOD. The health industry has done great work with soy products so make sure and check those out.   Slim Genics (http://www.slimgenics.com) has a huge line of healthy snacks as well.

During your Break Through weight loss journey, I'd avoid nuts because they are high in fat. Almonds and unsalted sunflower seeds would be okay but don't get hooked on that habit.

For other healthy diet snacks, consult your local nutrition store.

Sweeteners, Sauces, and Salt

I use sweeteners but in moderation. Specifically, I use Splenda and Stevia and only ½ of the small packets. Sometimes, I only use a third but don't use more than ½ a packet per cup of coffee.

Sauces and dressings are like mud. They slow down your body's ability to process the food they are covering up. If you must use a sauce or dressing, use a light version or even Fat-Free version. Just drizzle it over your salad instead of dumping it. I use about a table spoon on my salads and that is enough for me to get the taste mixed in well. When you eat at restaurants, make sure you order the dressing on the side.

Salt is also an important part of your Break Through weight loss. The amount of water you're drinking also washes away the salt that your body needs (and craves) so you'll need to add it back in. I use Morton's Lite Salt and nothing else. In the morning, I moderately salt my eggs and in the afternoon, I sometimes salt some celery to help curb being tired in the afternoon.

How to Handle the Mid-Afternoon Fog and Late-Night Cravings

I'm sure you've had those times in the mid-afternoon where you begin to feel lethargic, foggy and sleepy. Or you're watching TV and there is a sudden urge for buttery-salted popcorn and a Coke. Do not reach for the high-cal, high-sugar, high-everything energy drinks. I haven't done much research on them but I do know that there is a better way.

First, what causes the fog-time and cravings? While you are reducing your carb intake and losing weight — as you will be in your Break Through adventure — something called 'ketones' in your blood are elevated to compensate for the lack or reduction of carbohydrates. This is a natural process and one that is a defense mechanism. Your body then cries out for a quick-fix and that is when you normally hit the left-over bagels or brownies.

Here are 3 ways I keep a handle on the cravings:

1. Make sure you are drinking your water. When you feel a craving coming on, reach for the bottle not the bagel.
2. Take a pinch of lite salt and suck on it.

3. A dribble of honey on your finger also helps clear the fog.

The Importance of Grace Time

Grace is a gift that is given to someone without strings attached. While you need discipline to have your Break Through weight loss (see "Get Your Head On Straight" above), you also need to know that IT IS okay to go off of your plan occasionally. I call those times "Grace Time" and I choose to take them. Here's an example:

Last night I was out with a dear friend and had a few beers and "bar food." I knew that this morning my weight would be up a pound or two. But I was okay with that because I chose to enjoy my friends company and I chose to enjoy some of the less-healthy options. Just like you are choosing to get healthier through your Break Through weight loss adventure, you can choose to give yourself Grace when you think it's appropriate.

The reason I call it "Grace *Time*" is because it is only a moment or meal. It is not a day. After a while, you'll physically find that your body doesn't crave the less-healthy options anymore. You are reprogramming your body and mind to want the healthier foods and drinks. But to repeat, it is okay to give yourself Grace occasionally. It doesn't make you a failure. It doesn't make you a loser. Mentally and physically, it could be the best thing for you.

My only advice in "Grace Time" is to let one of your support people know just so they can help you get back on track if need be.

What To Do When You Eat Out

For me, I use the same eating patterns as I do when I'm at home. In fact, I bring the above information with me. On my phone, I have a document that lists recommended food for each of the 5 categories so I can easily reference it at restaurants.

Most restaurants have healthy options such as make-your-own items like salads, pizza's and burgers. For lunch, I usually have some sort of salad, less any bread-like items and fat-free dressing on the side.

My wife and I split meals when we go out as well. It saves money, food intake amounts and you actually get more food together than in a single portion.

Here is a list of some fast food joints at which I eat:

* *Taco Bell*: I love their Fresco menu. You can ask to skip the mayo and cheese on the items as well.

* *Jimmy Johns*:   Remember that their meats, like all others, are processed.   But once in a while is okay (remember Grace Time).   They do, what they call, an 'Un-which' which is simply a sandwich without bread.   They substitute fresh lettuce wraps. Try it. It's really good.

* *Chipotle*:   I usually get their chicken salad in a bowl with a small amount of brown rice pico de gallo and hot salsa.

Some other fast food places like McDonalds have healthier menu items.   I suggest NOT going into McDonalds but go through the drive through.   Why? Because once you smell their fries and Big Macs, it's game over.

Here are three websites that list food chains that have healthy options:

http://bit.ly/1dOb6hy

http://fitm.ag/21wPdo

http://fxn.ws/11uiVRH

Vitamins

Because much of the food we eat has been stripped of nutrients in favor of shelf life, I recommend taking a daily vitamin as well.   There are 4 vitamin groups that you should take every day.   The first one is a must.   The remaining are strongly suggested.

(Remember to check with your doctor before changing any medications or vitamin regiments.)

1. Multi-vitamin. Here is one company that has done an incredible amount of research and has come up with multivitamin suggestions. http://bit.ly/SDG6Z9

2. Calcium. Calcium helps keep our bones and teeth strong and our muscles and nervous system needs it for proper functioning.

3. Vitamin C+D. Both of these help with absorption of food and help in the breakdown of other chemicals in the body.

4. Omega-3's. Unless you eat fish every day, you won't be getting enough fatty acids found in Omega-3's. They help keep your brain, joints and other parts of your body lubricated and help facilitate smooth breakdown of foods.

Break Through Your Plateau

There will be times during this journey when you get "stuck" at a certain weight for a while. That is called a weight loss plateau and it happens for a variety of reasons based on your body chemistry. It is normal for almost everyone. If you look at my chart in the previous section, you can see my times of being on the plateau. For some it happens at the beginning of week two. For others it happens later. Be prepared. It will happen.

I have three suggestions for you to break through that plateau.

1. DO NOT let the frustration stop you from your goal. You will get through it. It will just take time. It may be a few days. It may even be a few weeks but you will begin to lose the weight again if you keep diligent. Remember to call 1-800-hiking-partners! (Obviously, this isn't an actual number but it helps you remember the importance of the people you've told about your journey.)

2. Adjust your meals by eliminating the starch, decreasing your fruit intake by one serving per day and increasing your vegetable intake by one serving per day. In essence, your daily intake would be 3 proteins, 2 fruits, 4 vegetables and your normal snacks.

3. Keep drinking your water!

Again, remember that 80% of weight loss and good health is nutrition and 20% is exercise. Don't use this as an excuse not to get out there and get moving! Movement is essential to healthy weight loss and maintenance! So make sure that you are spending a significant amount of effort and energy in eating right and eating a lot of the right things. Also remember that …

YOU CAN DO IT!

YOU CAN BREAK THROUGH!

Summary

This was a huge chapter! It is the most important Break Through step so make sure you have the information readily at hand. In this chapter, we talked about the important role that nutrition plays, not only in Break Through weight loss, but in maintaining your health.

There are 3 "Don'ts"
1) Don't skip a meal
2) Don't eat fake (processed) food
3) Don't skimp on the right food

The key rule in portions is:

"FIST SIZE IS THE RIGHT SIZE"

There are 5 components of a Break Through Weight Loss Meal:
1) Protein
2) Vegetable
3) Fruit
4) Starch
5) Liquids

A few other things we talked about. Make sure you snack, just make sure they are healthy type snacks interspersed throughout the day. We talked about what kind of sweeteners, sauces and salt. We also mentioned that mid-afternoon and late-night cravings are perfect times for fruit and vegetables. Often though, your body isn't hungry but thirsty. Try drinking water and wait 5 minutes to see what happens.

Remember to give yourself a little Grace. Grace Time refers to those meals or times that you choose to go off plan, recognizing that you aren't a bad person for doing so. Just don't make it a normal habit and ask your friends to help you get back on track.

Eating out can be done with a little pre-knowledge. Just implement the 5-elements of a Break Through weight loss meal and you'll be good.

Finally, don't forget the Vitamins!

Again, consult your medical professional before starting any major changes!

Break Through 4: Weigh Everyday

Ok, that last Break Through was a doozy but very important! In terms of sustainability, Break Through 4 is even more important than Break Through 3 for long lasting weight control and health.

Weigh Yourself Everyday... Throughout the day

Mentally, you need to see where you are on your weight journey down and then longer-term maintenance for important reasons.

For one, seeing your weight mentally gives you a reality check for good or for bad. When I see that I've lost that pound, it causes me to evaluate the day before and repeat it. When I see that I've gained, I evaluate why that might be. Usually it was because I didn't front load my day, drink my water or I took Grace Time and ate off-plan. But that's okay because I know that seeing where I'm at helps motivate me to stay on track.

Again, to the right is my weight daily chart from my Google doc.

As you can see, it is evident that I had a few Grace Times and hit a few plateaus. But I also had so great

7/1	231
7/2	231
7/3	229
7/4	226.6
7/5	225
7/6	224.6
7/7	222.6
7/8	221.6
7/9	222.2
7/10	221
7/11	220.8

drops as well! Google docs lets you take this information and create a chart to see as well. Pretty cool!

I suggest that when you are at the beginning of this journey that you weigh yourself throughout the day if you can. For me, I learned that I'm always the lightest in the morning, heaviest in the evening. I also learned that if I weigh myself right before I go to bed that I can take that weight and shave off 1.5 - 2 pounds to estimate my next morning weight.

Buy the right scale for you

For some people, they want to know their fat ratios, their height-weight comparison and lots of details about their health. For others, they simply want a dial to tell them their general weight range. I fall somewhere in the middle. I want to know what I weight to the .10 place.

I bought a digital, middle of the road, scale. You don't need the *fancy-shmacy* ones that costs you big bucks. I spent $35 on mine.

Put Your Scale In A Visible Place

You know the phrase "Out of sight; out of mind." This holds true for almost everything — even weighing yourself daily. We have ours in our bathroom under the vanity. Every time I'm in there, I see the scale. My curiosity always has me jump on the scale. You may not be so curious.

Tips

Here are some tips on weighing yourself everyday:

* Record your weight at the same time every day. For me, the weights I record are always at the beginning of the day, after my first 'bathroom go'.

* Weigh naked. You want to get an accurate weight so yes, go ahead and strip down.

* Weigh your clothes. If you don't want to strip down (or are too lazy to do that), weigh yourself naked one time, then put your pajama's on and weigh again. Subtract the two and you'll have your "clothes — weight." For me, I know that my pajama's weigh roughly one pound. So I jump on the scale in my pajama's and subtract one pound. No stripping for me. Remember …

YOU CAN DO IT!

YOU CAN BREAK THROUGH!

Summary

In this chapter, we emphasized the importance of weighing yourself everyday!

1. Buy the right scale for you.

2. Make sure you see it everyday.

3. Record your weight at the same time every day.

4. Get an accurate weight both with and without clothes.

Break Through 5: Celebrate Milestones

Moments in life are meant to be celebrated. Milestones mark progress and remembering them is important to the human existence.

A milestone is an event marking a significant change or stage in development. Your weight journey is something to celebrate. If you've read this far, you've already hit a milestone because there is something in your brain that is telling you "You Can Do This!"

What to Celebrate

Here's what I did. At the beginning of my 40 pound Break Through weight loss journey, I figured out a reasonable celebration plan. I knew that the first week would be both exhilarating and depressing. Losing weight quickly made me feel great but it was also tough to feel my body struggling to adjust to the changes. So here was my plan:

* Milestone 1: On day 3 of week 1, I celebrated this first milestone by going to see a movie, bringing my light crunchy snack with me and I had a Diet Sprite. At the end of the week, I had a light beer to celebrate. As you notice, this first week was not

based on my weight but my determination to begin the journey strong.

    * Future Milestones: After that first week, I changed from celebrating time to celebrating weight loss. Every 5 pounds, I celebrated. 225, I ate a small bowl of chips and salsa (my favorite by the way!) 220 I bought a new pair of pants.   215, 210, 200 etc. Each one I broke through, I did something 'different' or 'special' to remember my journey toward better health.

I'd also celebrate what I was *gaining*. For me, I felt better walking up the stairs.   I was gaining comfortability and confidence.

Remember, what you <u>gain</u> by what you <u>lose</u> is an important part of why you're doing what you're doing. Celebrate the fact that you're gaining confidence. Remember that you're gaining health.   These are important if not primary in your Break Through weight loss.

How to Celebrate

This will depend on you.   For me, I decided that I was not going to make all my celebrations about food. So I bought new clothes, I went to special events, and I enjoyed some extra entertainment.   Yes, there were times of eating something special as well, but I tried not to focus on food during the celebrations. I highly suggest this for you as well.

The Outcome of Celebration

First, the downside. Realize that celebration with food will slow down your weight loss but that's okay. You've been heavy for so long, and extra day or two is not a big deal.

In his book, "The 4 - Hour Body," (http://amzn.to/18XXlnZ) Tim Ferris says that each week he has a cheat day. I'm a spiritual person and I don't cheat. I call it a Grace Time as I mentioned earlier, because it is on this day that I give myself grace. I celebrate the freedom I have to make choices and realize that God still loves me. It is on this day that I'll have my beer (in moderation) and a Taco Bell Fresco Double-Decker (just one).

The bigger outcome of these kinds of celebrations, however is a positive one. Mentally, recognizing that you are making progress boosts your endorphins — the happy chemicals in the brain. They give you strength to venture into the next chapter and gives you something to shoot for. Celebrations are key to making progress. As a friend of mine told me …

"How do you know where you're going if you don't know where you've been?"

Summary

Celebrating your milestones are very important in your Break Through weight loss because they remind you that you can do it!

* Celebrate not only your weight loss but also your health gains.

* Don't just mark your milestones by eating food you've set aside for the journey. Celebrate with events, a moderate shopping spree or extra entertainment.

* Celebration is good for your attitude and will help propel you into the next chapter of health.

First Steps

In one of the Star Wars episodes, Luke Skywalker is learning to be a Jedi from Jedi Master Yoda. In the famous scene, Luke says he'll *try* to use his mind to lift his X-wing star fighter out of the mud. Yoda looks at him and sternly says, "Do or do not. There is no *try*."

If I could be Yoda and you could be Luke Skywalker, picture me saying the same thing to you. DO NOT go on this journey if you're simply going to TRY it. You have to be able to say, "I am going to do this" or else you'll quit and then be depressed because you feel like a failure.

Go back and re-read the chapter on Mentality. Get your determination on and join me in getting lighter!

First steps

1) Consult a doctor if you have health issues before beginning. I know it's redundant but I want to see you Break Through and with your doctors help, it will make your journey even better.

2) Assemble your team of hiking partners according to the earlier chapter.

Another thing you can do is use a website called www.FutureMe.org. It allows you to write an email to yourself to be delivered at a future date. Write down a bunch of motivational phrases and email them to yourself over the next month. Just that little boost could get you through a rough patch.

3) For one week, faithfully follow the water addition, vitamin addition and weighing yourself everyday. You should lose about 2-3 pound by day 3. Keep a journal of your 1st week journey. Remember that day 3 will be a tough day because your body will begin to realize you're wanting to make a change so it will push back. Push back harder. This is where you employ your hiking partners.

4) After that first few days, adjust your diet according to Break Through 3 and go forward!

Last Words

Anytime you do something new, there is a thrill and a fear that happens. I believe that you are going to succeed in your Break Through weight loss. Why do I believe this about you? Because you've come this far in the book. You wouldn't be interested or motivated to make your life better if you weren't still with me.

I must warn you that you are about to do something that your history, experience and personality isn't going to want you to do. People around you may even tell you that you can't do it. DON'T BELIEVE THEM!

If you've taken me seriously, you most likely have some ingrained habits and thinking patterns that will fight against your change. This is why you NEED hiking partners. If they are the right people, they will encourage you when you need it. I still need the encouragement of mine and you will need yours too.

Above all, constantly play out your life. Focus on what you will be GAINING not losing and don't be hard on yourself.

I'd love to hear about your journey! So shoot me an email at www.toddstocker.com and remember that

YOU CAN DO IT!
YOU CAN BREAK THROUGH!

Before You Leave!

I need your help. You may know others who would benefit from this information. If you feel strongly about the contributions this book made to your health efforts, please take a few seconds to post a 5 star review on Amazon. Very few people ever leave 5 star reviews. So it is a big deal if you do. Writing a 5 star review is like tipping me $25. I really appreciate the gesture. I feel like million bucks whenever I get a glowing review. Just click here and it will directly take you to the page:

http://amzn.to/GVK105

If you have any questions, please email me at www.ToddStocker.com. I can't guarantee I'll respond but I'll give it a shot. You can also connect with me on Facebook and Twitter:

Facebook: https://www.facebook.com/todd.stocker3

Twitter: https://twitter.com/todd_stocker

Peace!

Todd

<u>Y<small>OU CAN ALSO CHECK OUT MY OTHER BOOKS:</small></u>

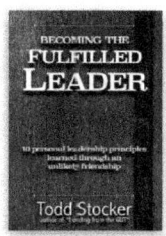

"BECOMING THE FULFILLED LEADER" — <u>http://</u>

<u>amzn.to/1wy43pE</u>

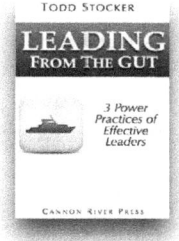

"LEADING FROM THE GUT" — <u>http://amzn.to/</u>

<u>1yRM1gn</u>

"ROSEMONT" — <u>http://amzn.to/16OK1vn</u>

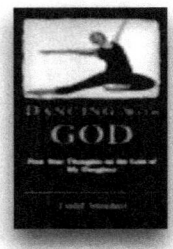

"DANCING WITH GOD - First Year Thoughts On The Loss Of My Daughter" — http://amzn.to/18L7riI

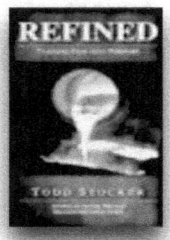

"REFINED - Turning Pain Into Purpose" — http://amzn.to/1ah7z8F

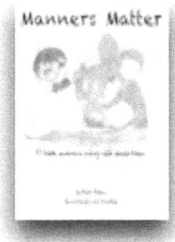

"MANNERS MATTER" — http://amzn.to/1glbkii

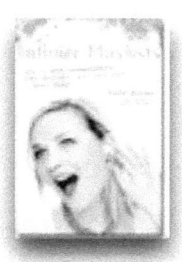

"INFINITE PLAYLISTS" — http://amzn.to/16u9bgL

Professional Partners

Below is a list of organizations that have helped me in my weight journey. I call them "partners" because in a sense, their services, expertise and information have helped me stay focused and achieve my goals.

    * Anytime Fitness - http://www.anytimefitness.com

    * SlimGenics - http://www.slimgenics.com/

    * WebMD Diet and Nutrition - http://www.webmd.com/diet/

    * Biggest Loser Nutrition - http://www.biggestloser.com/

    * The 10-minute Trainer - http://bit.ly/GCDtmU

    * Tim Ferriss - http://bit.ly/6YqX